MW01049519

This manual is written for patients with neck dis(... participants in a neck injury prevention program or for anyone who wants to have a healthy neck.

— H. Duane Saunders

SELF-HELP MANUAL

For Your Neck

by H. Duane Saunders, M.S., P.T.

Published by
The Saunders Group, Inc.
4250 Norex Drive
Chaska MN 55318-3047

612-368-9214 or 800-654-8357
Fax: 800-375-1119

Table of Contents

Edited by *Robin Saunders*
and *Beth Solheim*

Illustrated by *Mary Albury-Noyes*

Keylined by *Mary Schultz*

ISBN Number 0-9616461-3-6

copyright 1986, 1990, 1992
H. Duane Saunders

Introduction

There are no "magic answers" concerning the care of neck problems. Yet most neck problems are unnecessary and can be avoided. Years of experience show that patients are seldom cured of a neck problem with treatments such as manipulation, medication, traction, a neck brace, or surgery. Sometimes these treatments are necessary and effective, but what you do to help yourself is usually more important than what the medical practitioner does. For this reason, **For Your Neck** has been written to help you understand how you can have a healthy neck, or if a problem already exists, this self help manual will enable you to manage your problem more effectively.

Neck Pain is no joke! We are aware that pain affects each person differently and that some people do take advantage of workers compensation and sick leave by exaggerating or faking illness. When this happens, a company or supervisor may become suspicious of all workers who have neck and back problems. This leads to frustration and anger for everyone involved. We all must make an effort to be fair and honest when dealing with neck and back injuries and certainly recognize that most people are not faking or exaggerating their problems and pain.

It is important to understand that neck problems are seldom caused by a single injury. Most people think that their neck problems occurred at a particular time and place. This is almost always untrue! Neck problems often take months or even years to occur. A problem can be developing long before pain is noticed. Then, a sudden twist or stressful activity causes the pain to be noticed. This may cause the individual to think that something slipped out of place or was injured

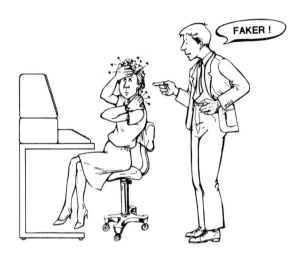

Neck pain is no joke.

at that moment. This is not the case, as it would take considerable physical injury for this to happen.

While it is true that some neck problems are the result of a single physical injury, most are the result of the cumulative effects of **poor posture, faulty body mechanics, stressful living and working habits, loss of flexibility and a general decline of physical fitness.** Most neck problems cannot be managed effectively unless these factors are recognized and dealt with.

Because of the long standing nature of many neck disorders, the problem may seem to be overwhelming. However, **the good news is that most neck problems are unnecessary and can be managed effectively. For Your Neck** demonstrates how.

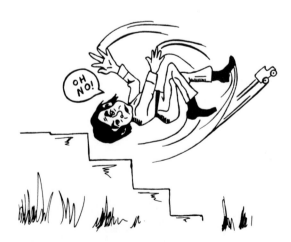

Neck problems are seldom caused by a single injury.

Anatomy

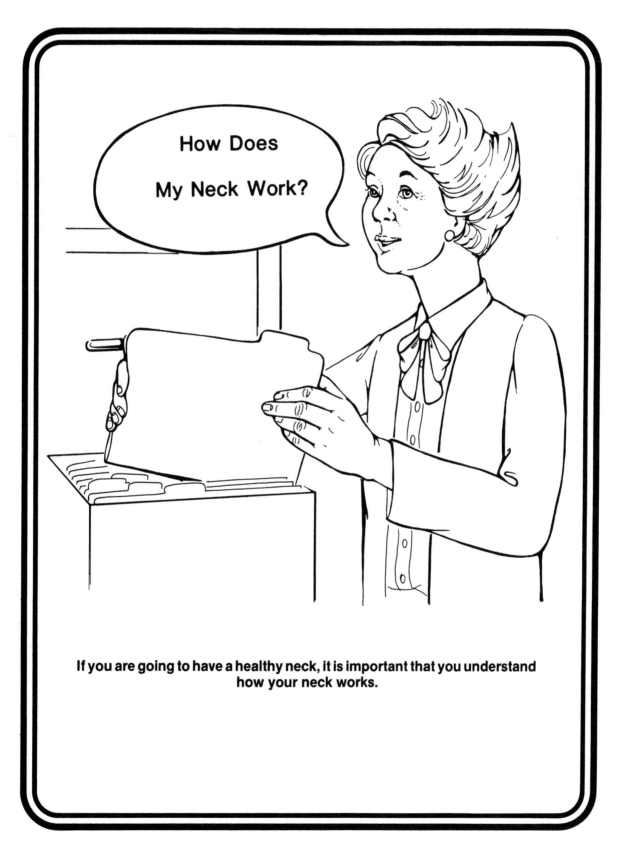

If you are going to have a healthy neck, it is important that you understand how your neck works.

The spine maintains the structure of our trunk and at the same time allows for flexibility and body mobility. It also provides protection for the spinal cord.

ANATOMY

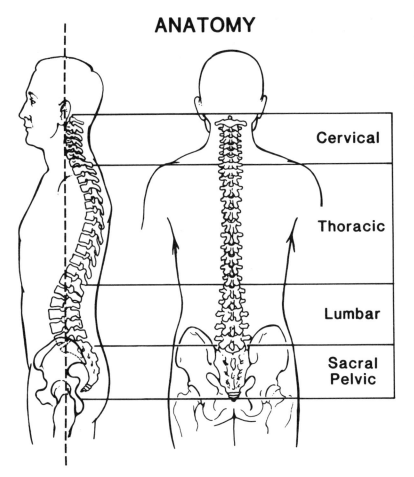

There are four areas of the spine. The cervical or neck region is made up of seven bones which are called vertebrae. This area is quite flexible.

The thoracic, or chest region, is made up of twelve vertebrae. There is generally less mobility in this region because the ribs attach to these vertebrae.

The lumbar or lower back region is made up of five vertebrae.

The sacral region is made up of one solid bone called the sacrum.

Notice that the spine is not straight. It is made up of four continuous curves. The neck and low back curves are concave to the back and the thoracic and sacral curves are concave to the front. These curves allow for flexibility and tend to help the spine in its role as a shock absorber.

One of the keys to having a healthy neck and back is maintaining the curves of the spine in a balanced position. When the spine is in this balanced position, weight is supported by the bones, and the muscles and ligaments are not under stress.

If the curves become either flattened or excessive, the balance and mobility of the spine may be altered and a disorder may eventually develop.

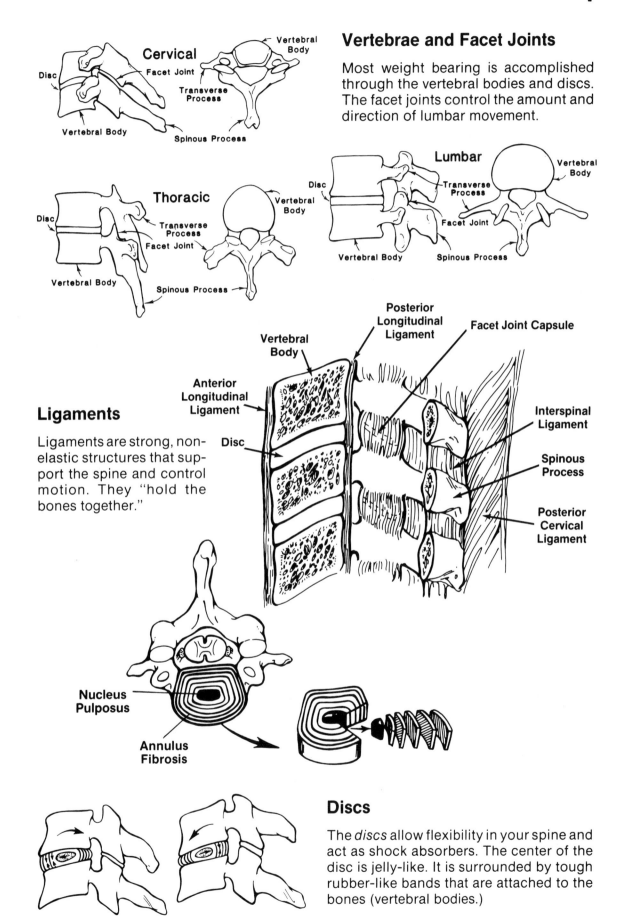

Vertebrae and Facet Joints

Most weight bearing is accomplished through the vertebral bodies and discs. The facet joints control the amount and direction of lumbar movement.

Cervical

Disc, Vertebral Body, Facet Joint, Transverse Process, Spinous Process, Vertebral Body

Thoracic

Disc, Vertebral Body, Transverse Process, Facet Joint, Spinous Process, Vertebral Body

Lumbar

Disc, Vertebral Body, Transverse Process, Facet Joint, Spinous Process, Vertebral Body

Ligaments

Ligaments are strong, non-elastic structures that support the spine and control motion. They "hold the bones together."

Vertebral Body, Posterior Longitudinal Ligament, Facet Joint Capsule, Anterior Longitudinal Ligament, Disc, Interspinal Ligament, Spinous Process, Posterior Cervical Ligament

Nucleus Pulposus, Annulus Fibrosis

Discs

The *discs* allow flexibility in your spine and act as shock absorbers. The center of the disc is jelly-like. It is surrounded by tough rubber-like bands that are attached to the bones (vertebral bodies.)

Nerves

The nerves from the spinal cord pass through openings between the vertebrae at each segmental level. The nerves in the neck supply the arms and the nerves in the lower back supply the legs.

There are two types of nerves.

Motor nerves carry impulses from the brain to the muscles. These impulses cause the muscles to contract and control movement of the body.

Sensory nerves send impulses from the body to the brain. Pain, touch, position, temperature, and other senses are felt through the sensory nerves.

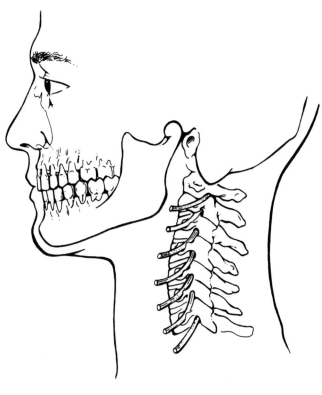

Muscles

There are many muscles that control the movement of the neck and upper back. The shorter, deep muscles control rotation or twisting. The superficial muscles are longer and control forward and backward bending and hold the spine upright.

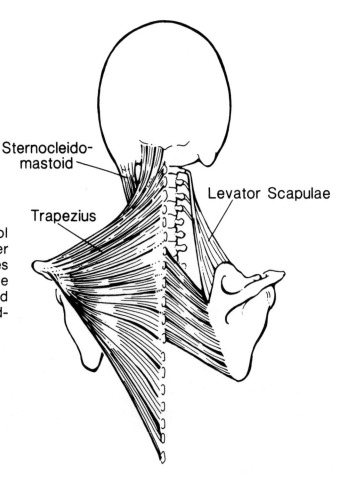

Sternocleido-mastoid

Levator Scapulae

Trapezius

Common Causes

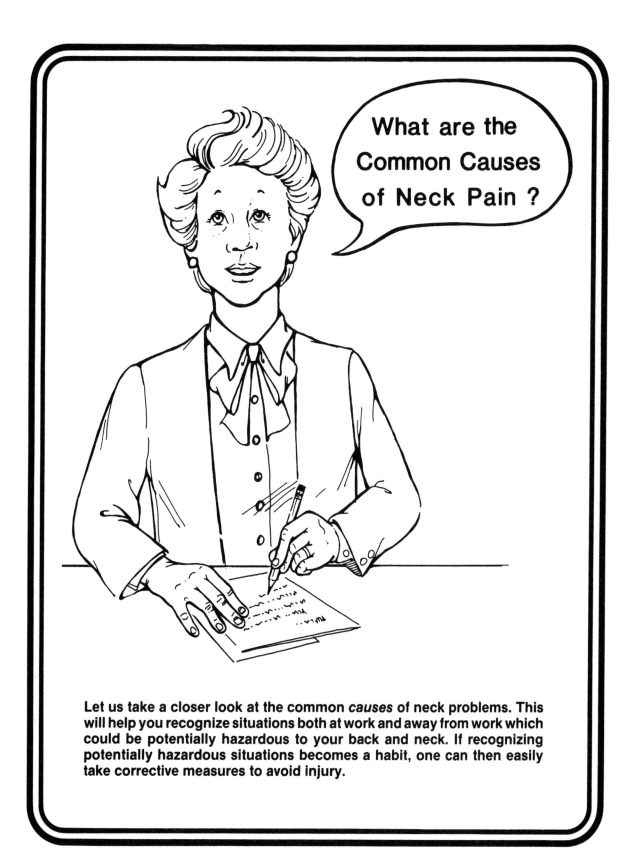

Let us take a closer look at the common *causes* of neck problems. This will help you recognize situations both at work and away from work which could be potentially hazardous to your back and neck. If recognizing potentially hazardous situations becomes a habit, one can then easily take corrective measures to avoid injury.

Common Causes of Neck Problems

Poor Posture

Poor posture is one of the leading causes of neck and upper back pain.

This is a common posture problem. With weak abdominal muscles, an increased curve or "sway back" may develop and cause a chronic strain on the facet joints and ligaments in the lower back. Sometimes, the forward head, rounded shoulder posture is associated with sway back. This causes increased stress across the upper back and base of the neck.

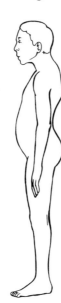

Flat back posture can develop because of bending and working in a stooped forward position too much of the time. We often see the forward head, round shoulders with this posture also.

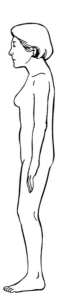

Avoid sitting with forward head and rounded shoulders. This is one of the leading causes of neck and back problems. Avoid all of the sitting postures shown here.

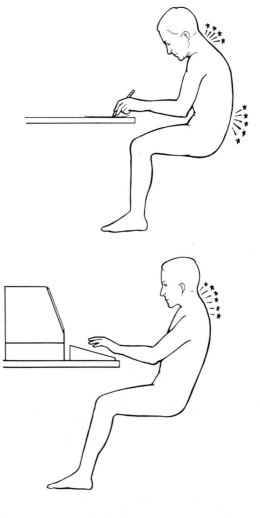

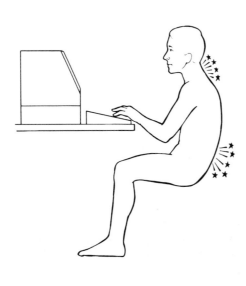

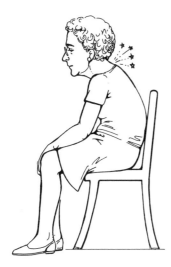

Studies have been done to measure the amount of stress placed at the base of the neck because of the forward head posture. It is estimated that there is as much as three times the normal stress and tension on the muscles and ligaments in the neck and upper back when the head is held 2 to 3 inches in front of the base of the neck and upper back.

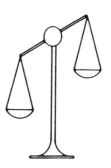

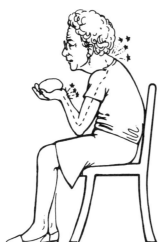

This can easily be demonstrated by holding a 10 lb. sand bag in one's hand as shown in this drawing. With the weight of the sand bag 2 to 3 inches in front of the wrist, one will soon feel the tension and stress develop. The same tension and stress can develop in the neck and upper back of a person with forward head posture.

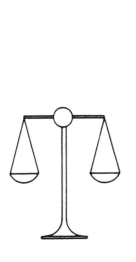

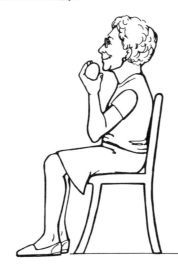

If the weight is brought back into alignment with the wrist, one can feel the tension and stress lessen immediately because now the boney structure of the arm is supporting the weight.

Good posture involves keeping the spine in a balanced position as much of the time as possible. It is when we move out of this balanced posture that we place stress on certain structures. It is especially stressful when the poor postural positions are maintained for long periods of time without change or interruption.

Common Causes of Neck Problems

Faulty Body Mechanics

Practicing good body mechanics is a 24 hour a day job. Poor posture and faulty habits have the same negative effects at home as on the job. Let us examine some unbalanced body positions that are common causes of neck strain during everyday activities. Many of them involve the slumped, forward head, rounded shoulder posture.

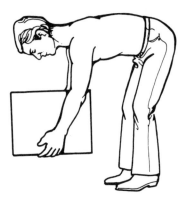

Don't lift with your neck and back flexed.

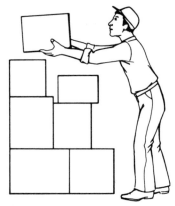

Don't lift with weight too far away.

Stressful Living and Working Habits

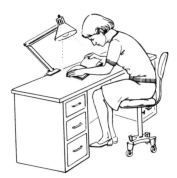

Don't lean over your desk or work for long periods of time.

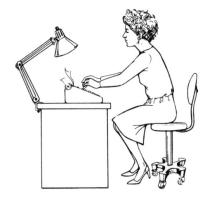

Don't sit too far away from your work.

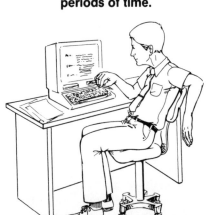

Don't lean away from your work while sitting. If you lean away from your work, you will have to bend your neck forward into a stressful position to see.

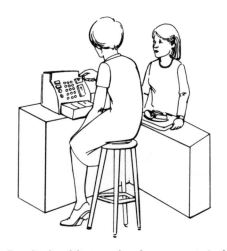

Don't sit with your back unsupported.

Stressful Living and Working Habits

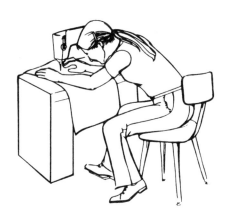

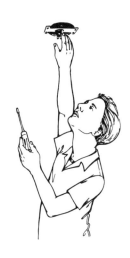

Don't work at a bench or table that is too low for you.

Be careful not to work overhead for long periods of time with your neck bent backwards.

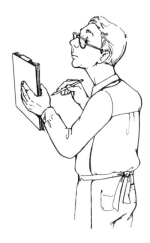

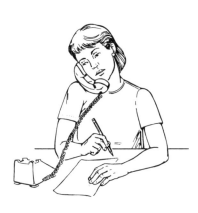

If you wear bifocal glasses, be careful not to thrust your head and neck forward when you read.

Don't twist your neck to hold the phone.

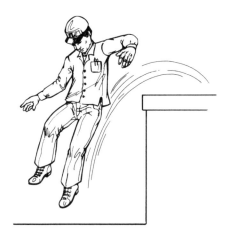

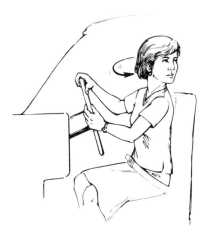

Don't jolt your spine unnecessarily by jumping out of your truck or off of a high object.

Don't just twist your neck to look behind you.

Just as you would not drive your car through every pothole in the road, don't subject your neck to unnecessary stress.

11

Common Causes of Neck Problems

Stressful Sleeping

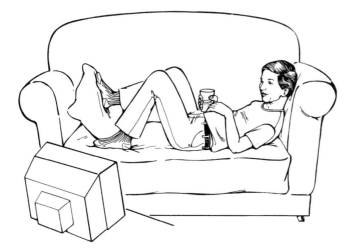

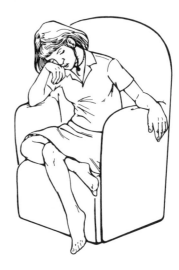

Don't lie in bed or on a sofa with your head propped up as shown in this slide.

Don't sleep in a chair without your head supported.

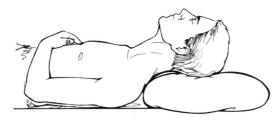

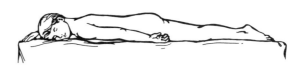

Don't use a solid foam rubber pillow; it is too firm and does not let your head sink in to give your neck the support it needs.

Don't use a pillow at all when sleeping on your stomach.

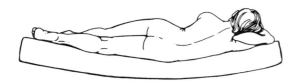

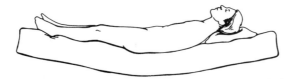

Don't sleep on a sagging mattress. Regardless of the position you sleep in, a sagging mattress will leave your back and neck in an "unbalanced" position.

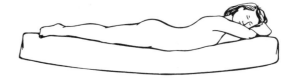

Loss of Flexibility

Loss of flexibility contributes to neck injury. The disc and facet joints in the neck and back do not have a blood supply. Nutrition is received through movement of body fluids into the disc and facet joints. If flexibility is lost, the nutritional supply is decreased to these structures. This permits weakening and makes them vulnerable to injury.

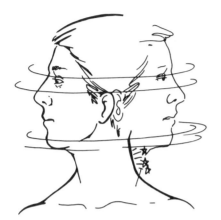
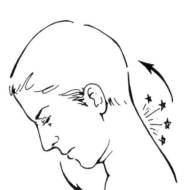
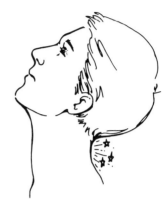

Decline of Physical Fitness

It has been shown that people in poor physical condition are much more vulnerable to neck and back injuries than those who maintain a high level of physical fitness.

Most jobs can be done without risk of injury if one is willing to maintain an adequate level of physical fitness.

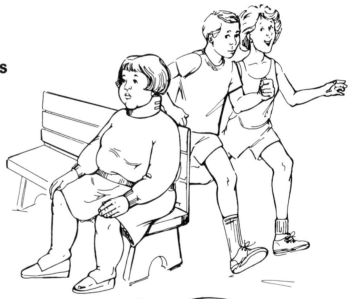

Accidents

We must also recognize that some neck injuries are caused by accidents such as falls, falling objects and especially automobile accidents . . .

. . . so we must follow safe living and working practices at all times.

Injuries caused by accidents will be much worse if one is in a general state of poor condition.

A healthy body can endure most stresses and strains without being injured.

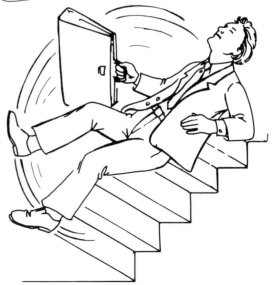

Common Causes of Neck Problems

Uncommon Causes of Back Problems:

1. Birth defects.

2. Metabolic changes or problems.

3. Infection

4. Tumors

5. Psychosomatic problems.

Also, stress, poor nutrition and smoking can make an already existing neck or back problem worse.

Remember . . .

Many people attempt to work at jobs that require considerable physical labor, but they do not keep themselves in the physical condition necessary to do these jobs. Companies can do many things to make the work place safer. However, a company cannot

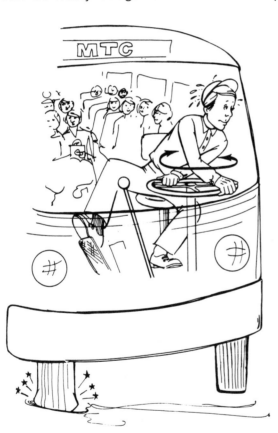

guarantee that all jobs will be totally free of activities and positions that contribute to neck injuries. Therefore, one must know how to maintain a healthy neck.

Many jobs will require some stressful positions and activities. Even when the work place is designed as safely as possible, these conditions will still exist.

However, stressful conditions will not lead to injury if one maintains good flexibility, a high level of physical fitness and if one practices good body mechanics and good posture whenever possible.

Common Neck Disorders

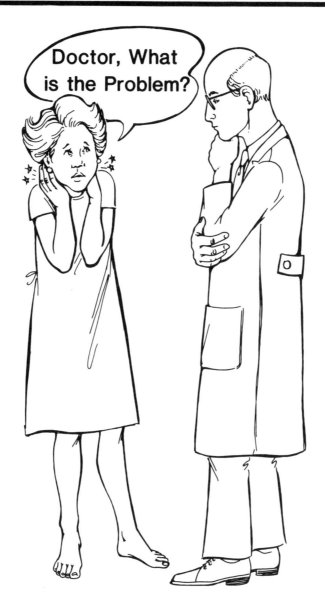

The most common neck disorders are:

1. Muscle spasm and inflammation.
2. Acute strains and sprains.
3. Chronic strains and sprains.
4. Joint stiffness.
5. Disc herniation or bulge.
6. Osteoarthritis.

In this section, the cause, pathology (description) and treatment of these disorders will be discussed.

Common Neck Disorders

Muscle Spasm and Inflammation

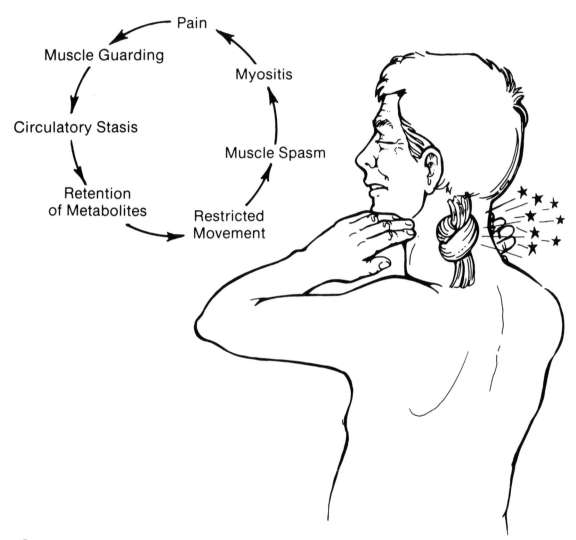

Cause

Whenever you feel pain of any kind, your body's first reaction is muscle guarding. The muscles "splint" or immobilize the area where you feel the pain. Prolonged muscle guarding produces muscle spasm and inflammation. Muscle spasm may be very painful but it is not necessarily a sign of a serious problem.

Pathology

Tender, painful muscle, slowed circulation and low-grade inflammation.

Treatment

This cycle often needs to be interrupted with medication and treatments such as heat, cold, massage or electrical stimulation. This treatment is often important and necessary, but it is doing very little to address the real cause of the problem.

16

Acute Strains and Sprains

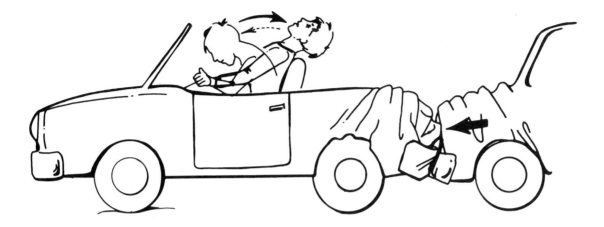

Cause

Acute injuries result from auto crashes, falls, falling objects or other traumatic accidents.

Pathology

There is often overstretching, tearing, bleeding and irritation of the muscle and ligament fibers.

Treatment

If the injury is minor, a few days of rest and avoidance of further aggravation is usually satisfactory. If the injury is severe, considerable time may be required for healing. During the healing period, muscles will often become weaker, joints will stiffen and poor posture will develop. This resulting problem must be corrected with gradual reconditioning to restore full flexibility, strength and good posture. The help of your doctor or physical therapist may be necessary. Healing of the injury will probably occur regardless of what you do following this type of injury; **reconditioning** is the most important thing to remember.

Chronic Strains and Sprains

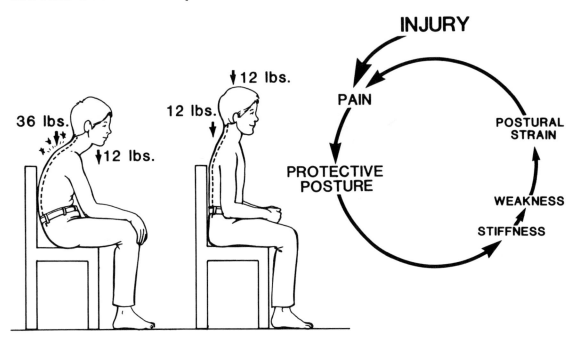

Cause

Chronic strain often develops following acute injuries because flexibility, strength and good posture were not restored. Neck strain is a good example. Because of pain one tends to hold the head and neck in a slumped protective posture during the acute injury stage. As healing takes place, the ligaments and muscles adapt to the new position. This eventually causes pain because of the strain of the abnormal posture and the loss of flexibility. Chronic strain can also develop because of poor posture and faulty work habits. In fact, postural strain related to the slumped sitting, forward head posture is a leading cause of headaches, neck and upper back pain.

Pathology

Overstretching and/or irritation of the individual muscle and ligament fibers.

Treatment

General strengthening and flexibility exercises are helpful but, most importantly, you should learn to correct the posture that is causing chronic pain. Changing positions frequently is helpful. Perhaps you need to change your work or home environment. Often an exercise program that stresses general fitness such as walking, swimming, bicycling or sports is helpful.

Joint Stiffness

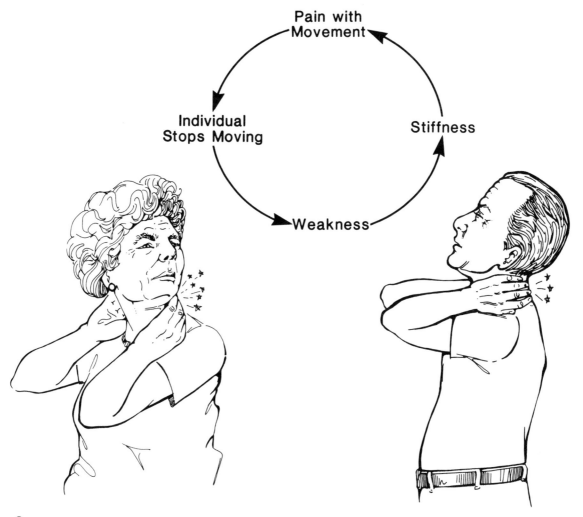

Cause

Joint stiffness may result following healing of an injury, may occur because of poor posture or may be the result of inactivity and a sedentary lifestyle. Thus, a vicious cycle occurs. When stiffness develops the individual feels pain and he or she moves less and less to avoid the pain. This causes more weakness and stiffness to develop which in turn actually makes the pain worse. This sequence of events often occurs with individuals who are genuinely interested in recovery. It may even happen because of the advice of a medical practitioner.

Pathology

The ligaments around the joints become thick and inflexible. When attempts are made to move the joint, pain results. The stiffness retards circulation to the joint, causing degeneration of the structures.

Treatment

Flexibility and stretching exercises and correction of faulty posture are the main things one can do to treat joint stiffness. A regular exercise program and return to a more active lifestyle is often helpful. Your medical practitioner can give you advice.

Disc Herniation or Bulge

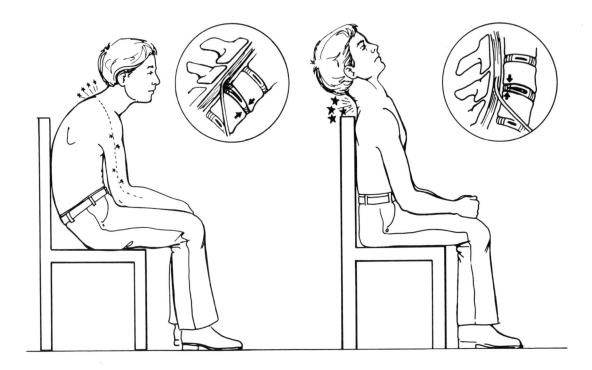

Cause

The most common cause of a bulging disc is sitting in a forward slumped position too much of the time. It is almost never the result of one injury and usually takes months or years to develop. Loss of flexibility and poor physical fitness are almost always related causes.

Pathology

The jelly-like center of the intervertebral disc is squeezed through the cartilage rings causing the outer wall of the disc to bulge. This puts pressure on the nerves in the disc wall which send neck and arm pain messages to the brain. In some cases, numbness, weakness and reflex changes occur in the arm.

Treatment

Proper treatment consists of correcting the faulty habits and posture which caused the problem. Backward bending flexibility must also be regained and proper balanced posture maintained until the disc has a chance to heal in its proper position. Traction and a neck support are necessary in some severe cases. Surgery is sometimes necessary. In most cases, a small disc bulge can be prevented and/or corrected by backward bending and avoiding forward bending and slumped sitting for awhile. However, a word of caution: if this backward bending exercise causes increased *arm pain,* one should *stop.* Some *neck pain* with this exercise is *ok.*

Osteoarthritis

Cause

Osteoarthritis is simply the wearing out of the joints in the neck. It occurs in everyone to some extent as he or she becomes older. It is due to degenerative or "wear and tear" changes that occur in our daily lives. Osteoarthritis sometimes occurs as the end result of long standing neck problems related to sprains, strains and disc injuries, as well as to repeated wear and tear. In other words, degenerative changes may gradually develop after one has experienced repeated injury or incidence of a neck problem.

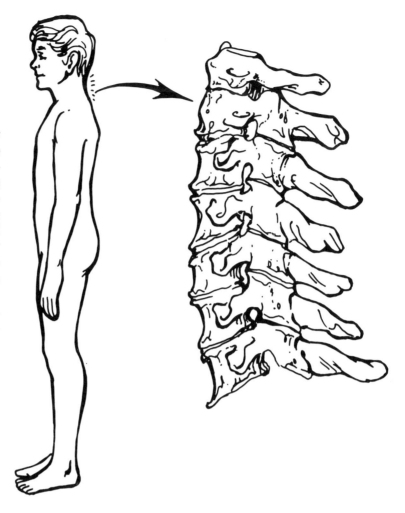

Pathology

Osteoarthritis may involve a wearing out and narrowing of the disc, roughening of the facet joint surfaces, thickening of the joint capsule and ligaments and narrowing of the opening for the spinal nerves. In severe cases, the nerve may be irritated or "pinched" because of this narrowed opening.

Treatment

Even though this disorder seems as though it would be serious and would cause a lot of problems, we know that many people have osteoarthritis of the spine and actually have very little, if any, pain and discomfort. Many people become alarmed when they find out that they have osteoarthritis in their necks or backs. This is unfortunate, because such a condition does not necessarily mean that one is going to have pain.

People who have degenerative arthritis in the joints in their necks and backs should exercise regularly and try to maintain a reasonable level of flexibility and physical fitness. Use common sense and follow the advice of your **medical practitioner.**

On the other hand, overexertion and certain physical activities may aggravate this condition and one should learn to avoid the specific activities that seem to be stressful. Later you will learn six simple rules to follow when exercising which will help you decide what is best for you.

Other much less common neck disorders include:

Facet joint locking

The joints catch and lock in one position.

Joint instability

Can result from overstretching or torn ligaments (as in whiplash.)

Traumatic fractures

Rare, but serious result of an accident (a broken vertebra.)

Stress fractures

Very rarely occur as a result of repeated stress on the spine.

Compression fractures

Occur in older people (especially women) as a result of inactivity and metabolic changes. (Mostly in mid-back area)

Tumors

Very rare; may occur in someone who has had previous cancer.

Disease and illness elsewhere in the body

Sometimes such things as kidney or prostate infections or meningitis cause back pain.

Emotional stress brought on by worrying, or holding back feelings, can cause muscle tension and aggravation and may magnify an existing problem. The nervous, tense person may take longer to recover from an illness or injury.

Treatment

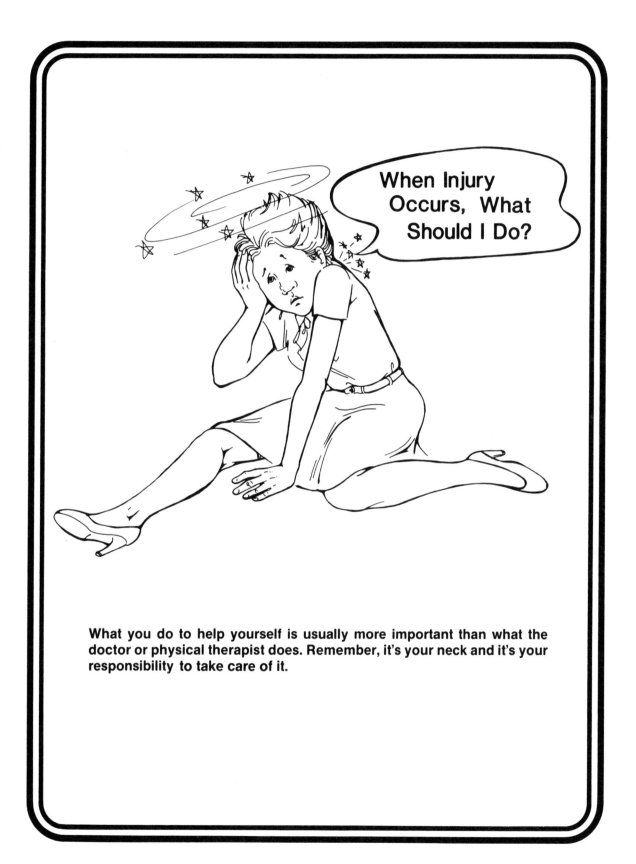

What you do to help yourself is usually more important than what the doctor or physical therapist does. Remember, it's your neck and it's your responsibility to take care of it.

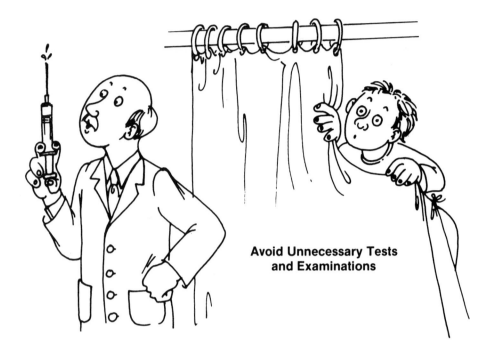

Avoid Unnecessary Tests and Examinations

Evaluation — The Exam

Most physicians and therapists go through most of the steps mentioned here. Shortcuts must be avoided, but it is important to remember that each examiner will do things a little differently.

1. A complete history, which will frequently include the following questions: How did your pain first start? What was the exact position you were in when you were injured? What is the exact location of your pain? Does coughing or sneezing make it worse? What makes it better? What previous treatment have you received?

2. Physical examination to determine the following: Your general posture, muscle tone and range of motion; areas of local tenderness and muscle spasm; and possible muscular weakness and sensory changes in the extremities.

3. A physician may also want to use special studies such as laboratory tests, x-rays, myelograms and CAT scans to identify the extent of a disc problem or an electromyogram to identify nerve damage caused by a "pinched nerve". Although these tests are sometimes needed, in most cases they are unnecessary and should only be done when a severe problem is suspected or when standard, more conservative treatment doesn't seem to be helping.

IF SEVERE INJURY HAS OCCURRED

If severe injury has occurred, **see your doctor.** He or she will examine you to rule out serious injury such as a fracture. **Ice** is often helpful in reducing internal swelling, pain and muscle guarding. It is important to **rest** the injured area and avoid aggravating it further. A soft collar or other type of neck **support** may be helpful.

AS ONE BEGINS TO IMPROVE

As one begins to improve, **careful movement and exercise** should be started. Flexibility and strength should be restored as healing takes place and a normal, **balanced posture** should be maintained throughout the course of recovery.

THE ULTIMATE TREATMENT

The ultimate treatment for most neck problems is **eliminating the cause.** Medications are sometimes helpful in reducing pain, muscle guarding and inflammation, but they actually do very little or nothing to correct the disorder itself. Physical therapy treatments are sometimes used to relieve the pain and muscle guarding, and certain treatments such as traction are given to help correct the actual problem.

Rest and relaxation are also important in recovery. In addition to eliminating the cause of the problem, **exercise to restore strength, flexibility and fitness is the answer.**

RETURN TO WORK

In some cases, return to work after an injury may need to be gradual. Many companies have implemented light duty or part-time jobs for a short time, especially when the worker's regular job requires considerable physical labor and/or stressful activities.

25

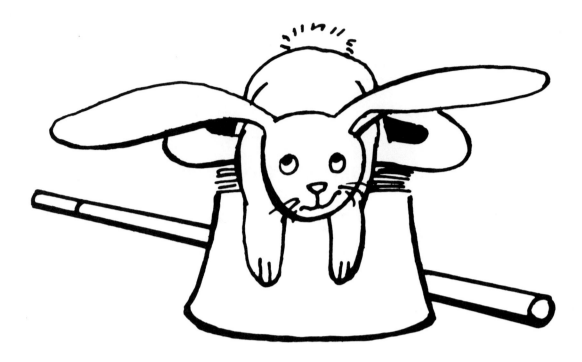

Stop looking for Magic Answers.

In most cases the individual is ultimately the only one who can effect a cure for a back or neck problem. What you do to help yourself is usually more important than what the doctor does. There are times, however, when it is essential for you to seek medical help for a neck or back problem. When a severe injury is involved, if there is weakness or numbness in your arm or leg, or when a problem is persistent and does not respond to common sense management, you should follow the advice of your medical practitioner.

How many times have we seen newspapers, magazines and television depicting another "magic answer" for the treatment of a neck or back problem? It seems that as soon as one "magic answer" is proven to be ineffective, another takes its place.

Some medical practitioners seem to encourage this passive attitude as if there is a magic "pill", "pop", "twist", "stretch" or "surgery" that will cure the problem. While there is often a place for many of these treatments, they should not be looked upon as "magic" cures. Ultimately you are responsible for your own cure.

Neck Care

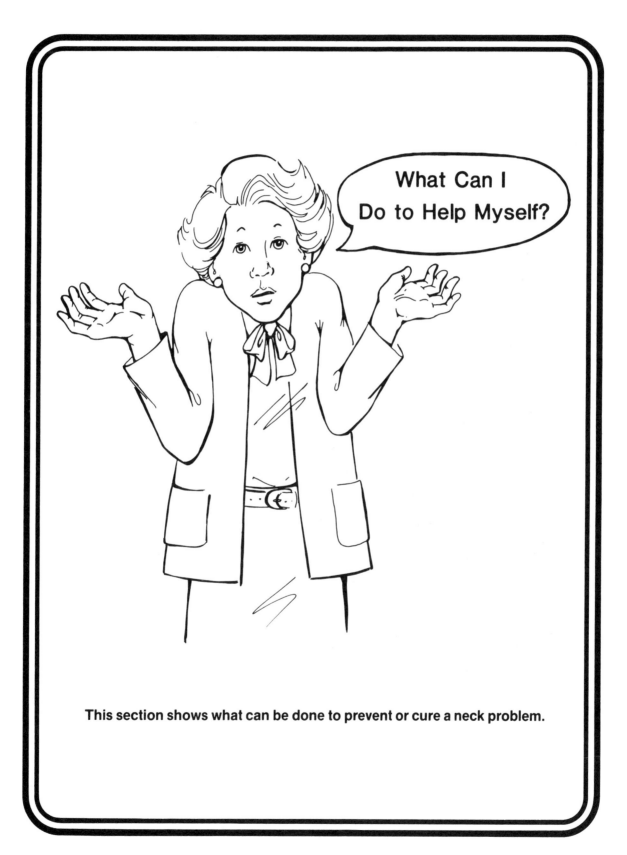

This section shows what can be done to prevent or cure a neck problem.

Neck Care

Posture

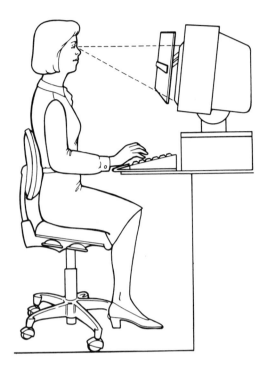 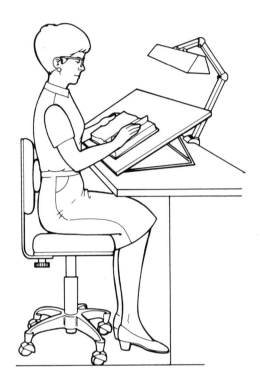

Sitting** — **Proper sitting posture is one of the best things you can do to prevent back and neck problems.

Bring your work close to you and raise it to the right height whenever possible. The right work height depends on the task you are doing. In computerized office work places, raise the height of your monitor so the top of your screen is about eye level and position hard copy at the same distance and tilt as the monitor.

When reading or performing desk work consider an inclined work surface. The inclined surface helps to reduce unnecessary bending of the neck and back while helping to keep the shoulders back and out of a rounded posture.

It is often helpful to place a rolled towel or small pillow or cushion behind the lower back to maintain the normal arched position. The position of the lower back is important in maintaining correct positioning of the neck as well. In fact, the forward head, rounded shoulder posture almost always accompanies a slumped lower back; so remember, good posture starts at the lower back. A variety of cushions and back supports are available for office chairs and automobile and truck seats.

If you must work for extended periods with your arms away from the sides of your body, chairs or work surfaces with arm rests are helpful to support the weight of the arms. If you do a lot of sitting at your work, seek alternate ways to do some of your work. If you spend a good deal of time on the telephone, consider using a headset.

28

Posture

CORRECT SITTING POSTURE

- Head and shoulders erect and balanced.
- Close to the work.
- Back supported in natural curve.
- Arms at sides.

- Feet flat on floor or foot rest.
- Hip/trunk angle > 90°.
- Even weight on buttocks and thighs.
- Freedom to move.

What to look for in a chair:
1. Hydraulic controls
2. Seat back adjusts up/down
3. Seat back pivots forward/backward
4. Seat pan tilts
5. Five caster-easy roll base
6. Seatback supports natural lumbar curve
7. Seat height adjusts
8. Waterfall seat front
9. Seat back and seat pan appropriate size for user

Additional features when needed:
- Arm rests
- Stool height with foot rests
- Self locking casters
- Material/fabric appropriate for environment
- Casters for carpeted versus vinyl floor

Posture

Standing — Good balance is the primary goal.

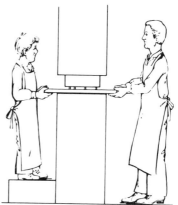

When standing keep work at a proper height so the neck and lower back are held in an upright, balanced position. Over the past 100 years, the average height of individuals has increased several inches.

Because of this, many current work stations have been designed too low, especially for taller individual. It may be wise for companies to consider work stations of adjustable height when possible, or to raise the work height of fixed equipment. A shorter person can usually stand on a platform or stool if the work height is too high, but there is nothing that can be done for the taller worker if the work station is too low.

Work Height

The right work height depends on the task you are doing. You can easily determine the right work height: For regular work, position the hands at about elbow height, for light assembly or precision work, your hands should be 4 to 6 inches above elbow height and for heavier, more forceful, work or work which requires downward pressure, your hands should be 4 to 6 inches below elbow height.

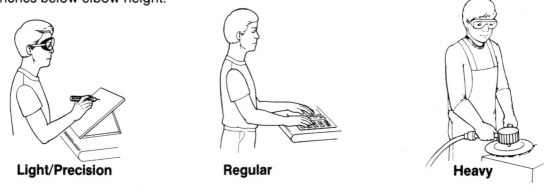

Light/Precision   **Regular**   **Heavy**

Working overhead with the neck and head bent backward for long periods of time is stressful. Use a step stool or ladder to bring yourself up to your work when possible.

Arrange shelves so that the heavier, more frequently used items are between shoulder and waist height, which is a more convenient height for lifting. The lighter, less frequently used items are placed higher, and the items which are rarely used are on the lower shelves.

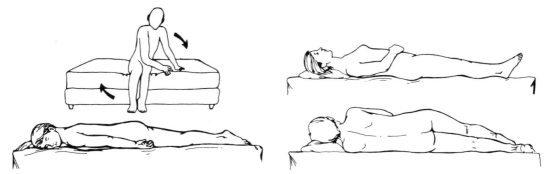

Sleeping — Sleeping on your stomach is not necessarily bad for you. There is no best position. You will probably find the one that's right for you.

One should sleep in a "balanced position". This means a firm support that is soft enough on the surface to accommodate the normal curvatures of the body.

Ideally, your pillow should support your head and neck in a neutral position. This means that most of the support should be under your neck, not your head. If you use a regular pillow, it should be made of feathers or fiber, not foam rubber, as foam does not mold to the shape of your neck; it bounces back. There are, however, a variety of foam rubber pillows contoured especially for the neck which have proven beneficial for certain people with neck problems.

While sleeping, it is best to change positions frequently. A king or queen size bed is often helpful because it allows more freedom to move and change positions.

Waterbeds are often recommended for persons with back problems, but experience has shown that they are not beneficial for everyone. When a waterbed is used it should be kept relatively full of water to maintain a firm foundation of support. Sleeping on the stomach is not necessarily bad positioning. A pillow is not recommended while sleeping on your stomach.

Body Mechanics

The most important principle to remember when lifting is to keep the head upright and the back in an arched position. This arched position tends to put the muscles in a shortened and strengthened position. It also distributes the weight more evenly between the disc and the facet joints, and it places a more balanced weight on the disc.

It is often helpful to place one foot ahead of the other in order to get the object being lifted closer to the body. This is especially important when lifting large, bulky items. This diagonal lifting position also balances the weight within a wide, safe base of support.

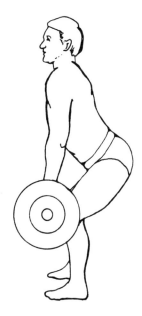

Keep Back Arched When Lifting

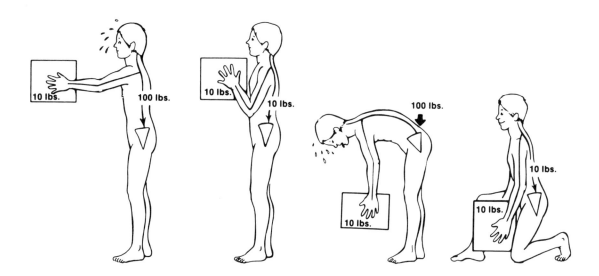

Keep Weight Close to Body

It is essential to keep weight close to the body. A ten pound weight held at arm's length increases the load by as much as seven to ten times the actual weight of the object. If the weight is held close to the body, there is not a great increase in the amount of stress on the lower back. And remember, activities which are stressful to the lower back are almost always bad for the neck too.

Body Mechanics

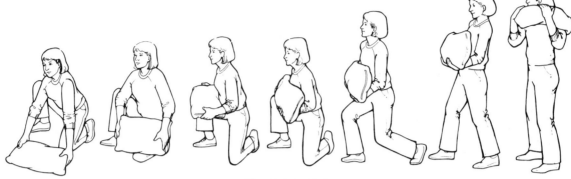

The Tripod Lift

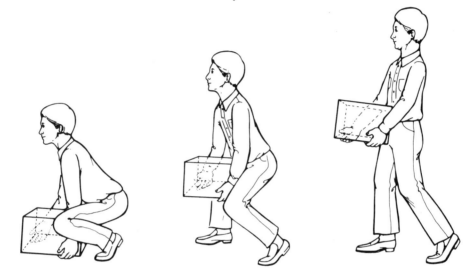

The Diagonal Lift
Squat, Head Up, Back Arched, Feet Spread One Foot Ahead As You Lift.

With heavy or bulky items, more than one person may be required or a mechanical hoist or lifting device may need to be used. Injuries often occur in industry as the result of forward bending and lifting when mechanical lifting devices are readily available, but are not used.

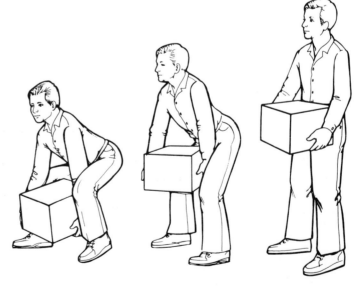

The Power Lift
Partial Squat, Head Up, Back Arched,
Feet Spread One Foot Ahead As You Lift.

Interrupt or Change Stressful Positions Frequently

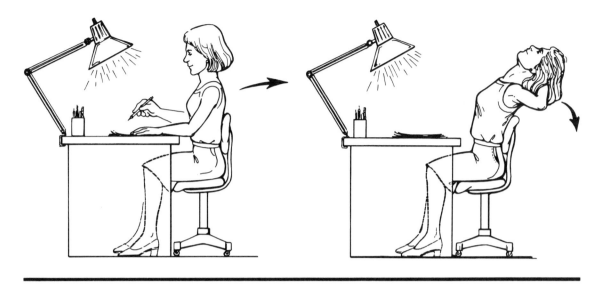

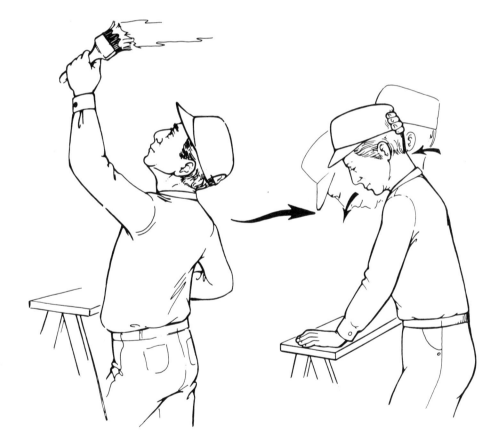

Interrupt or reverse stressful positions often. This is one of the key points of THE NECK CARE PROGRAM.

Many jobs require stressful positions and activities, but if they are interrupted frequently, injury will be prevented.

33

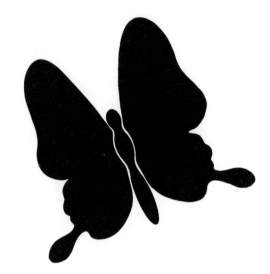

People who are emotionally upset or who are under a lot of stress will have greater difficulty with neck pain and headaches. Regular rest and relaxation is essential. Constructive problem solving may be needed in some cases.

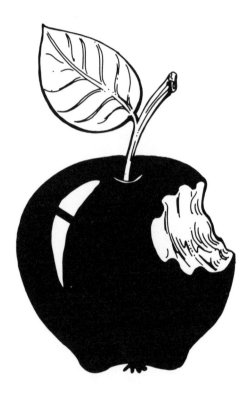

Nutrition plays an important part in our general health and affects the way our body heals when injured. Therefore, your diet is another important factor to consider if you want to have a healthy body. To do this you must take an interest in learning about good nutrition and good eating habits and discipline yourself accordingly.

Stop Smoking

Recent clinical studies show a direct relationship between smoking cigarettes and occurrance of neck and back problems. Smoking also restricts circulation and slows down healing when an injury occurs.

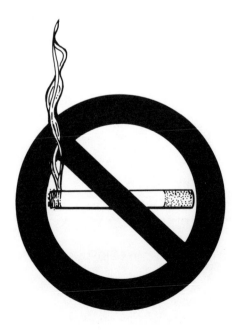

Exercises

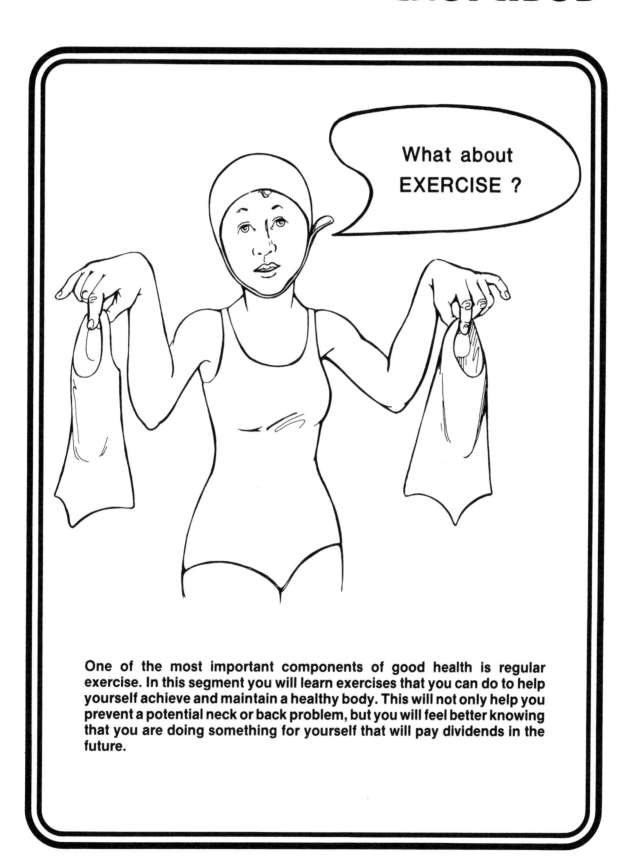

One of the most important components of good health is regular exercise. In this segment you will learn exercises that you can do to help yourself achieve and maintain a healthy body. This will not only help you prevent a potential neck or back problem, but you will feel better knowing that you are doing something for yourself that will pay dividends in the future.

A Full Physical Fitness Program

We know that exercising regularly promotes cardiovascular fitness and reduces the risk of certain diseases. Exercise also promotes mental well-being. Many people exercise in order to look slim and trim, while others exercise to develop strength and flexibility to help them become better athletes.

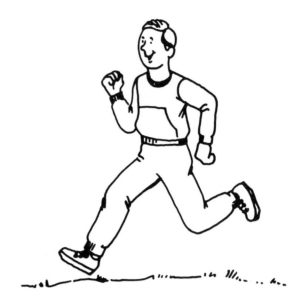

While the list of reasons to exercise is a long one and you should not need further motivation, we want to give you one more reason. Exercise regularly so you can live your life free of neck and back pain.

There is considerable evidence to support the fact that regular exercise is the single most important thing that you can do to have a healthy neck and back.

So you see that the most important exercise program one can do is to maintain a regular physical fitness program.

Rules for Exercise

- Exercises should be done **regularly.**

- Always **start out mildly** and **increase gradually.**

- **A little pain with exercise is usually normal,** but **exercise should not cause pain that lingers after you have stopped exercising,** and exercises for the neck or back should not cause arm or leg pain.

There are four basic types of exercise:

- **aerobic**

- **strengthening**

- **flexibility**

- **relaxation**

Aerobic Exercises

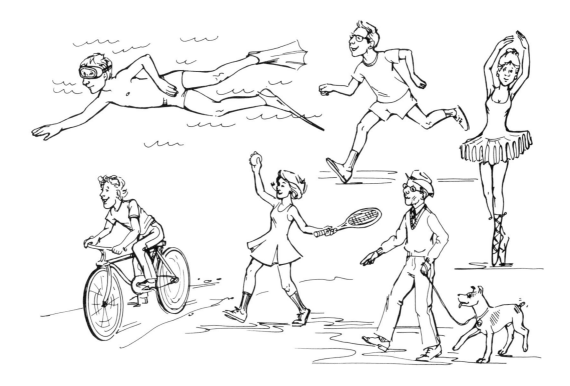

Aerobic exercises cause increased heart and lung activity and are done to improve cardiovascular fitness. Rhythmic, repetitive, dynamic activities such as running, bicycling, swimming, and walking that are sustained over a sufficiently long period of time, usually 20 to 30 minutes, are considered aerobic exercises.

Although one normally thinks of aerobic exercises as being beneficial for the heart and lungs, studies show that individuals who are in good cardiovascular shape are less likely to suffer from neck and back injuries. Therefore, the benefit of this type of exercise cannot be overlooked if you want to have a healthy neck and back.

Running, walking, swimming, bicycling and sports activities are all good for the neck and back if approached in a common sense manner.

For an exercise to be aerobic, heart and breathing rate must be increased to an exercise level. As a general rule, a recommended exercise heart rate is 220 – age × .7. If you are 40 years old, that would be 220 – 40 = 180 × .7 = 126. Another way of judging if an activity is within the aerobic exercise range is to notice a definite increase in breathing rate but at the same time still be able to carry on a conversation without difficulty.

Flexibility Exercises

Earlier we learned that joint stiffness and loss of flexibility is a common cause of neck pain. Therefore, **flexibility exercises** are important for many. If a joint or muscle is stiff, pain will be felt at the limit of range of motion. This is not the case when a muscle or joint has normal flexibility. Therefore, one of the signs of joint or muscle stiffness is limited range of movement and pain at the end of the range.

"A good rule of thumb" is this: If you have limited movement and some pain is felt at the end of that movement, you will need to do flexibility exercises. If you seem to have full movement and no pain is felt, you probably do not need to do that particular flexibility exercise.

It is important to follow this rule because it is <u>possible to be too flexible.</u> Joints and muscles can be overstretched. Unfortunately, some athletes and exercise fanatics spend too much effort stretching. Weakened joints and muscles are the result. If you are not sure which exercises you should do, or how vigorous you should be, your physical therapist or doctor can advise you.

The following flexibility exercises for the neck and upper back should first be done as a test. If you feel stiffness as you do certain exercises, you will want to include these in your regular exercise program.

Forward head, slumped sitting posture involves rounding of the shoulders and upper back. The muscles and ligaments in the front of the chest and shoulders may become tight with this type of posture.

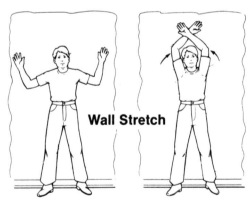

Wall Stretch

The wall stretch is done by standing with your back against the wall as you turn your arms out and raise overhead. Keep upper arms and body in contact with the wall as you do this exercise.

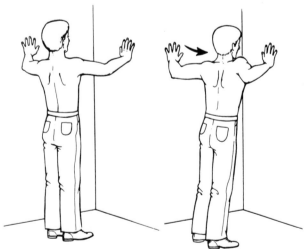

Corner Stretch

This exercise stretches the chest and shoulder muscles and ligaments. It should be held at least 15 to 20 seconds. Repeat the exercise a few times with hands at different heights until you feel you have gained flexibility.

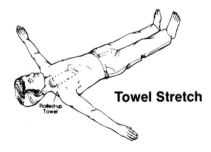

Rolled-up Towel

Towel Stretch

Another chest and shoulder stretch is done by lying over a towel roll as shown here. You may maintain this type of stretch for 3 to 5 minutes.

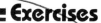

Flexibility Exercises

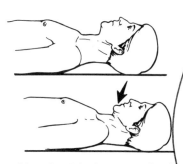

The head back, chin in, exercise is excellent for stretching tight muscles and ligaments in the back of the neck. Initially, the exercise can be done lying down, as shown . . . . .

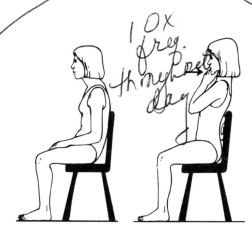

. . . . . and advanced to the sitting or standing position as you make progress. If you work with your head and neck in a forward bent position it is good to do this exercise frequently to relieve stress and tension.

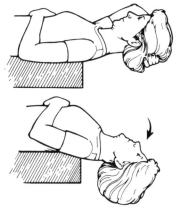

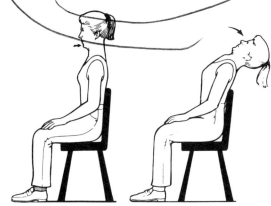

Backward Bending with Chin Tuck

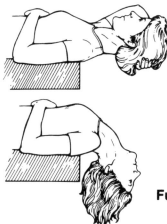

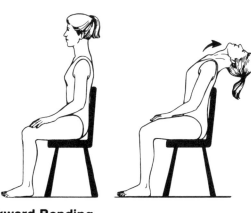

Full Backward Bending

Backward bending of the neck and upper back is especially helpful if you feel stiffness across the upper back and base of the neck. Start doing this exercise lying down as shown here, lowering the head slowly with your hand . . . . .

. . . . . and progress to the sitting position as you become more advanced. This is another excellent exercise for you to do frequently throughout the day if the forward bent head and neck position is a necessary part of your work. To concentrate the stretch to the upper back and lower neck, only do it with a chin tuck.

Exercises

Flexibility Exercises

The range of motion exercise shown here are important if you are limited in neck rotation.

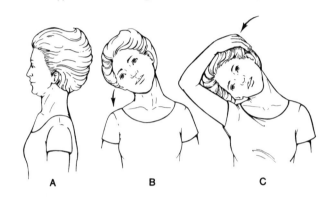

A   B   C

Side bending range of motion is shown here. Make sure the chin is tucked with this exercise.

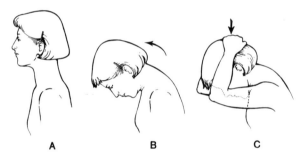

A   B   C

Forward bending range of motion is shown here. Notice that if an additional stretch is needed it can be applied with your hands with all of these exercises.

A   B   C

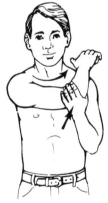

The middle-upper back stretch is done by gently pulling the elbow toward the opposite shoulder as shown here.

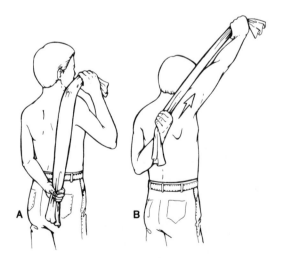

A   B

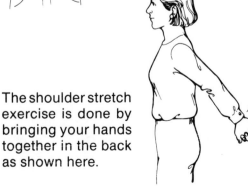

The shoulder stretch exercise is done by bringing your hands together in the back as shown here.

The internal rotation shoulder stretch is done with a towel as shown above.

Strengthening Exercises

To maintain good posture and have a healthy neck and back you must have good, well balanced muscular strength. Even some people who exercise regularly do not develop balanced muscle strength.

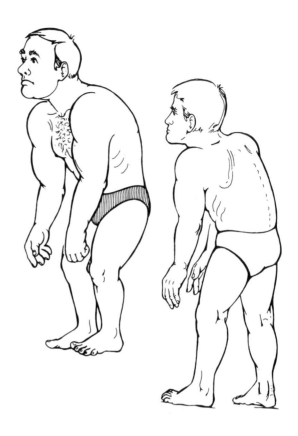

For example, a weight lifter may concentrate solely on chest and arm **strengthening exercises** and neglect strengthening exercises for the upper back muscles. The stronger chest muscles will pull the shoulders forward causing a rounded shoulder posture and a strain on the ligaments and muscles of the upper back.

For strengthening exercises to be effective, the muscles must become fatigued while exercising. This increased work load causes the muscle to grow stronger. If your muscles are weak, only mild exercise will be needed to fatigue the muscle. As you grow stronger, more repetition or resistance must be added to work the muscle enough to make it grow even stronger.

Generally speaking, exercises utilizing heavy resistance and fewer repetitions build power, or muscle bulk, while exercising with mild resistance and greater repetitions build endurance.

Power is needed for heavy work activities and certain sports. Endurance is more important for good posture and most of our everyday working and living activities.

Resistance may be added to most exercises in the form of free weights, exercise machines or elastic stretch material such as rubber tubing. Sometimes just working against gravity is enough resistance.

Although it is often desirable, it is not necessary to move through full range of joint movement for strengthening exercises to be effective. If moving through full range of movement with a strengthening exercise causes discomfort or aggravation, it should be modified by shortening the arc or range of motion.

Aerobic exercises such as walking, swimming and bicycling are also important general strengthening exercises. The following exercises are more specific for strengthening the upper back and chest, shoulder and neck.

Remember each of these exercises should be started mildly; you may gradually increase resistance and repetition as you grow stronger.

Exercises

Strengthening Exercises

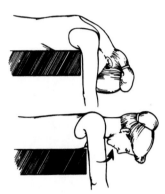

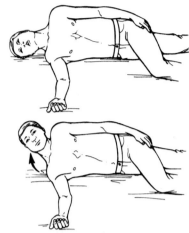

The head back, chin in, exercise that was shown earlier as a flexibility exercise, is also a strengthening exercise, especially if done against the resistance of gravity as shown here.

This side lying exercise is an especially effective neck strengthening exercise. A small pillow can be placed under the head to shorten the range of motion of this exercise if movement through full range of motion causes aggravation.

Isometric neck strengthening exercises are done by applying resistance with your hands to prevent movement as you contract the muscles. Continue breathing normally during all isometric contractions. Isometric exercises should be done for a 5 to 10 second hold. Isometric exercises do cause some compression of the joints and discs in the neck and may aggravate certain conditions.

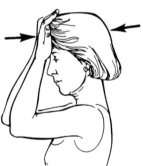

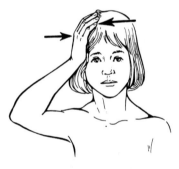

An isometric exercise to strengthen the front neck muscles is shown here. Press your forehead into your palms, but do not allow any motion.

An isometric exercise to strengthen the side neck muscles is shown here. Press your hand against the side of your head. Try to bring your head to the side, but resist any motion.

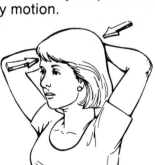

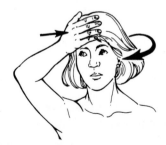

An isometric exercise to strengthen the muscles in the back of the neck is shown here. Press both hands against the back of your head. Try to pull your head back, but resist the motion.

Isometric rotation is shown here. Press your hand against your temple. Try to turn your chin to your shoulder, but resist any motion.

Strengthening Exercises

A very effective way to strengthen the neck muscles is with elastic tubing attached to a head band. The resistance can be varied from very light to very heavy depending on the size of the tubing and the tension applied. These exercises can be done in rotation, side bending, forward bending and backward bending.

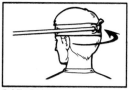
ROTATION

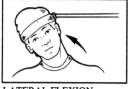
LATERAL FLEXION

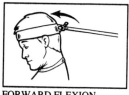
FORWARD FLEXION

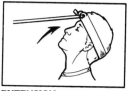
EXTENSION

An effective exercise to straighten the front neck and chest muscles as well as the abdominal muscles is the partial sit-up.

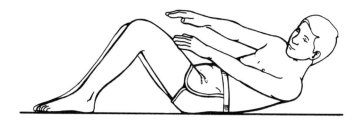

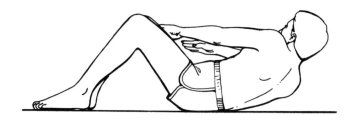

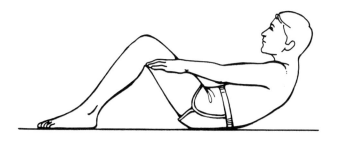

Partial sit-ups are done correctly with the hips and knees slightly bent. One should raise the arms, head and shoulders off the floor as shown. The position is held for five to ten seconds. One should raise to the point that the lower back is lifted from the floor. The feet should not be stabilized, because this allows the leg muscles to do the work and lessens the effectiveness of the abdominal muscle strengthening. The partial sit-up should be done with a slight right and left twist to strengthen the oblique muscles of the abdomen.

43

Strengthening Exercises

There are several exercises that will strengthen the back muscles. If you do a lot of sitting or forward bending, these exercises will be especially beneficial. The head should be supported in a neutral position as you do these exercises.

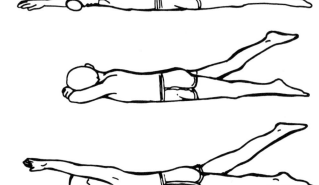

Single and double arm raises are especially effective for strengthening the upper back.

Leg raises strengthen the hips and lower back. Remember, good neck and upper back posture starts by sitting and standing with a strong, balanced position of the lower back.

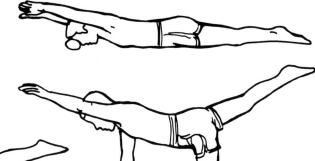

As you advance with these back strengthening exercises, progress to the alternate arm, leg exercises as shown here. Small ankle and wrist weights can be added to make these exercises more advanced.

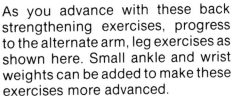

The exercises shown here are effective for strengthening the upper back and shoulder muscles.

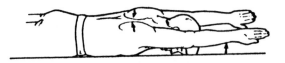

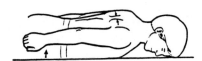

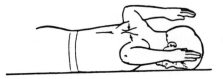

44

Strengthening Exercises

Exercises utilizing rubber tubing for resistance are very effective for strengthening the upper back and shoulder muscles.

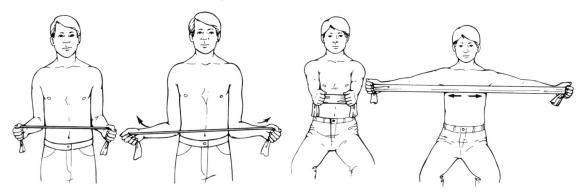

The exercise shown here strengthens outward rotation of the shoulder.

This horizontal pull exercise strengthens the muscles that retract the shoulder blades. This exercise, combined with the outward shoulder rotation exercise shown previously, is especially effective if you have slumped, rounded shoulder posture.

This exercise strengthens the front of the shoulder and chest muscles. Anchor or loop the rubber tubing around something stable. Position yourself so you are pulling your hand toward your abdomen against resistance. Keep your elbow bent to 90 degrees and against your side.

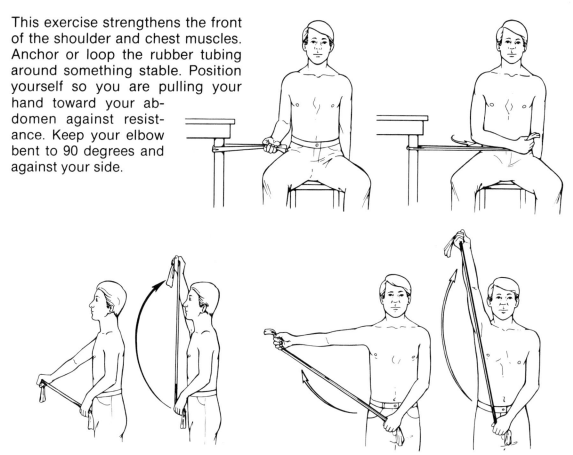

Shoulder strengthening exercises are shown here. Anchor the rubber tubing at your hip with one hand as you pull against resistance out to the side and overhead and out to the front and overhead. Keep the elbow straight as you do this exercise.

Relaxation Exercises

Relaxation exercises are important, especially if you have to spend a lot of time in one position without moving for long periods of time. They help to counteract the tendency to develop tight, sore muscles because of prolonged sitting or standing in undesirable postures.

Shoulder shrugs are done by pulling the shoulders up, causing a strong contraction of the neck and upper back muscles. The contraction is held for a 5 to 10 second count, then completely relaxed. Breathe deeply and slowly and feel the tension leave the muscles. This exercise can be done sitting, standing or lying down.

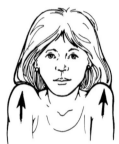

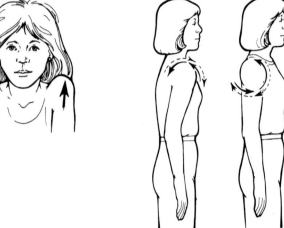

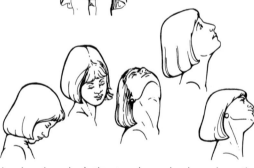

Interlace your fingers. Lift your arms up over your head as shown. Press your arms backward as far as you can. Then lean side to side to stretch and relax the muscles of the trunk and upper back.

Shoulder rolling is done by pulling the shoulders back, then up, forward and down in a circular motion. Roll several times in one direction, then reverse and roll several times in the opposite direction.

Head and neck circles are done slowly and gently in one direction, then the other. Repeat several times.

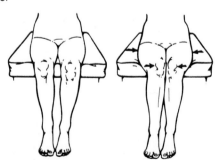

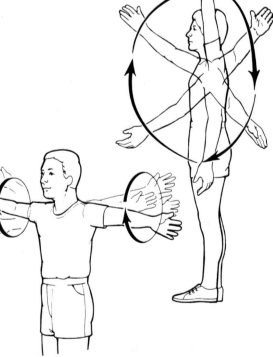

While lying or sitting quietly, practice tensing the muscles in a part of your body such as your hands, thighs or shoulders. Hold the contraction for a few seconds, then consciously allow the muscles to relax. With concentration and practice, you will learn to control muscular tension.

Arm circles are an excellent way to relax the neck and upper back muscles. Raise your arms straight out to the side. Slowly rotate your arms in small, then large circles forward, then backward.

FOREARM STRETCH (extensors)

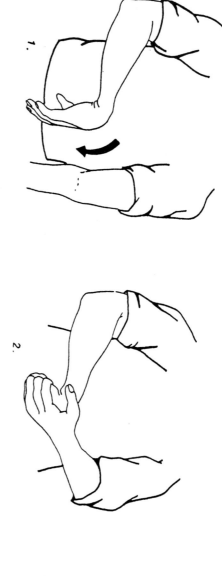

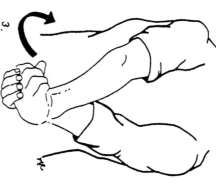

1.) With elbow bent and hand positioned close to chest, bend wrist and point fingers to floor.

2.) Use the other hand to keep the wrist bent while you straighten the arm in front of the body.

3.) The hand and forearm should rotate so that the palm is facing up. Attempt to bend the wrist more with the other hand. Hold for 10 seconds. Change hands. Repeat 3 times.

Median nerve stretch

Stand perpendicular to wall

HAND on WALL

Shoulder at 90°

Elbow straight

HANO flat on wall

Hold for 20-30 seconds. Complete 5-10 reps. Several times throughout day.

* Less of stretch - hand higher on wall

Be sure that you stand up straight with shoulders back.

Best time to do a stretch is in the shower or right out of shower. Moist heat helps tendons/muscles/nerves become more flexible.

- If painful at wrists, ice for 20 minutes.

"Never ice then stretch".

If pain & numbness persists — wear resting splints at night.

If muscular tension is a problem for you, you owe it to yourself to take the time to practice these techniques to allow yourself to relax. Many of the exercises shown earlier such as the head back, chin in, exercise and the isometric neck strengthening exercises are also effective relaxation exercises. Any exercise that requires a muscle contraction followed by a conscious relaxation effort has a relaxing effect. In fact, any physical activity, exercise or movement has the potential to relieve muscular tension. Your body was made for movement. Change or interrupt your body positions frequently. Find different positions in which you do your work. This, combined with a regular exercise program and making a conscious effort to relax, will help free you of muscular tension pain and headaches.

Ideally, one should set aside a specific time each day to exercise. However, when this is not possible, one should remember that many exercises can be done throughout the day. When you have a few spare minutes, take the opportunity to stretch, or do one or two of the exercises in your program.

Remember, the Rules of Exercise:

1. **Exercise should be done regularly.**

2. **Always start out mildly.**

3. **Increase the intensity gradually.**

4. **A little pain during exercise is OK.**

5. **Exercise should not cause pain that lingers.**

6. **Neck exercises that cause arm pain or back exercises that cause leg pain should not be done.**

LAST WORDS!

It is true that many of us work hard at our jobs and it is sometimes difficult to think that we should exercise when we are already tired from work. However, you should remember that hard work and exercise are not always accomplishing the same thing. In most work situations, we get too much of one type of activity or exercise and usually not enough of another.

Many people work hard all day, yet are still very stiff and are in poor cardiovascular condition. An exercise program should emphasize the type of exercise that is lacking at work. For example, if one spends a lot of time bending forward at work, he or she should emphasize backward bending exercises at home.

WCC 3